Why are we getting sick?

Robert S Cushenberry

DEDICATION

I WOULD LIKETO THANK MY WIFE DINAH FOR HER
TREMENDOUS SUPPORT AND LOVE SHE GAVE ME
DURING THIS VENTURE. WITHOUT HER INSIGHT,
ENCORAGEMNT, AND WISDOM, I WOULD HAVE NOT
COMPLETED THIS TASK.

FINALLY TO ALL THE READERS OF THIS BOOK, I HOPE
YOU FIND THE COURAGE TO MAKE CHANGES IN YOUR
LIFE AND THE LIFE OF YOUR FAMILIES. WE ARE TRULY
IN A BATTLE FOR OUR HEALTH

Cover pictures used with permission from Dr. Gilles-Eric Séralini

This book is my opinion and is for educational purposes only. It is not intended change anyone's life style. It is not intended to treat or diagnose any disease. I have been a medical professional for over 27 years and I have seen a disturbing increase in diseases and death. There are many people and corporations who disagree with me.

During my research I discovered a common link to the increase in illness. So I will share my findings with you. You must decide if you and your family's health are worth fighting for.

Based on my experience and research we are intentionally being poisoned by for profit corporations and our government is ok with it. Corporations have a legal mandate to make a profit with no concern for our health or the earth. Food corporations are no different than other corporations when it comes to profit

Toxic Poisons in our environment

Toxins are intentionally being placed in our food, water and everyday products we use in our homes. Sadly, our children and elderly are the most vulnerable. Your babies are being damaged before they are born. With so much working against us it's a wonder more people are not sick. Our bodies have become a dumping ground for disease causing toxins.

Every day we are ingesting genetically modified foods, MSG, Aspartame, Fluoride, pesticides, and antibiotics in meat. It's no surprise we are seeing an increase rare diseases, cancers and neurological problems.

Mother's your babies are being exposed to harmful ingredients in your womb. Aspartame, Dyes, MSG, and Preservatives are crossing the placenta lodging in your un-born baby's' brain and causing many health and behavior problems later in life.

Many of the cosmetics we use every day are known to have cancer causing ingredients in them. There is no real control or testing of cosmetics done on humans. Yet many of the ingredients are known to cause serious health problems in animals.

The EPA and FDA allow corporations to add tons of known harmful toxic chemicals into our food and water in the name of good taste and profit. Some countries have outlawed the use of these same toxic chemicals added to our food here in the United States. More cancers, tumors and chronic illness are on the rise as more and more chemicals are intentionally added to our food and water.

CONTENTS

ACKNOWLEDGMENTS

So you want to know the truth about good health! Our good health is being undermined by large for profit corporations, FDA, EPA, large food companies and drug companies. A new government health mandate is totally against good health and our choice to receive the health care we want.

The government wants our health and medical history. The ultimate goal is to put computer chips in all of us. The chip will be needed to receive medical and health care.

The FDA will collect our DNA for the federal government. Our health is now more at risk more than ever before. Huge profits, greed, and people control are the driving forces to steal your health.

Good health is a matter of life and death. Remember the saying "what you don't know won't hurt you", well that's not true. What you read here will shock and surprise you. Sometimes knowledge can be very disturbing especially when it affects our well-being.

What I'm going to share with you is public information. The knowledge we need is often intentionally hidden from us. We are in a battle for our good health, but most of us don't know it.

Chapter 1
WHAT IS GENETIC ENGINEERING/ GMO?

Genetic engineering involves laboratory techniques used to isolate and combine the genetic material of any species, and then to reproduce them in cultures of bacteria and viruses in the laboratory.

Unrelated genes are being mixed.

These techniques allow genetic material to be transferred between species that would never mix in nature. Human genes are placed into pigs, sheep, fish and bacteria; and spider silk genes in goats. Completely new, genes are also being introduced into our food and other crops. Genetic engineered foods are dangerous and the unknown consequences will be manifested in nature and in our bodies. Scientists have opened Pandora's box and released Franken foods into our food chain and there is no turning back, we and our children are the Guinea Pigs.

Genetic-engineered-foods have genes and parts of DNA from other species put into them. GE provides a set of techniques to cut DNA at will from specific sites. The different segments of DNA can be reproduced and stuck next to any other DNA of another cell or organism.

Species barrier

Genetic engineering makes it possible to break through the species barrier and to switch information between unrelated species. Genetic engineers are now splicing the anti-freeze gene from flounder into tomatoes and strawberries. A toxic gene from bacteria which kills insects is placed into corn, cotton and rape seed. Human genes are placed into pigs to produce Human Growth Hormone to produce faster growth in pig.

Overcoming species barriers

In order to overcome natural species barriers limiting gene transfer and maintenance, genetic engineers have made variety of artificial vectors (carriers of genes) by combining parts of the most infectious natural vectors – viruses, and plasmids.

These artificial vectors generally have their disease-causing functions removed or disabled, but are designed to cross many species barriers, so the same vector may now transfer, human genes spliced into the vector, to the genomes of all other mammals and plants on the earth.

Promoter Switch

The promoter switch is genetic material that is attached to the foreign gene before it is inserted into the host. Cells have evolved a defense system to protect the DNA from foreign invaders. Cell's don't know what to do with a gene it has never seen before. Should it be turned off or turned on? The new gene is given a Promoter Switch (aka light switch) which keeps all the cells in a permanent on position.

Virus Genetic Invaders

Certain Viruses have highly aggressive genetic invaders which gets past a cell's defenses and some are cancer causing. Viruses have evolved very powerful promoters which command the host cell to produce viral proteins.

The Cauliflower Mosaic Virus

The Cauliflower Mosaic Virus (CaMV) promoter is designed to overcome plant cell defenses, which prevent the foreign DNA from being expressed. The Cauliflower Mosaic Virus promoter enables the virus to overcome a plant cell's genetic operation and make copies of it. By overcoming the cell DNA defenses the CaMV operates independently of the cell's self- regulation and cause the gene to switch into overdrive.

The plant has no say in the expression of the new gene. CaMV is closely related to human hepatitis B virus. The new gene can end up anywhere, next to any gene or even within another gene, disturbing its functions. If the new gene gets into a dormant non-expressed area of the cell's DNA, it will interfere with the regulation of gene. It can cause genes in the dormant DNA to start producing proteins against the wishes of the cell.

How Are Genes Transferred?

There are different ways to get a gene from one species to another species. A vector is something that can carry the gene into the nucleus of a host cell. Vectors are commonly bacterial plasmids or viruses. The shotgun method, is when tiny gold particles coated with the new gene is shot into a plate of plant cells, hoping to hit somewhere in the cell's DNA.

Plasmids can be found in many bacteria and are small rings of DNA with a limited number of genes. Plasmids self-replicate and are easily reproduced and passed around.

The genes and gene-constructs created in genetic engineering have never existed in nature. They consist of genetic material from bacteria, viruses and other genetic parasites that cause diseases and spread drug and antibiotic resistance genes. They are designed to cross all species barriers and to invade genomes. The spread of such genes and gene-constructs have the potential to make infectious diseases untreatable and to create new viruses and bacteria that cause diseases.

Bacteria can exchange genes across species barriers in nature three ways.

(1) Conjugation is where genetic material is passed between cells.

(2) Transduction is when genetic material is carried from one cell to another by infectious viruses.

(3)Transformation is the process by which genetic material is taken up directly by the cell from its environment.

Genetic parasites, viruses, plasmids and transposons, have special genetic signals to escape being broken down. A virus consists of genetic material usually wrapped in a protein coat. After entering a cell and shedding its protein coat, the genetic parasites can hi-jack the cell and make more copies of it. Plasmids are pieces of free, usually circular, genetic material that can be maintained in the cell separately from the cell's genome.

Transposons, or jumping genes, are blocks of genetic material which have the ability to jump in and out of genomes, with or without multiplying themselves in the process.

What is Horizontal gene transfer?

Horizontal gene transfer is the transfer of genetic material between cells of unrelated species, by processes other than usual reproduction. During the usual process of reproduction, genes are transferred vertically from parent to offspring; within a species or between closely related species.

What are the dangers of horizontal gene transfer?

- Heart disease, arrhythmia
- Leukemia
- Thyroid suppression
- Tumor Growth

- Infantile acute leukemia
- Osteoporosis
- Thyroid damage
- Increased Cancer Cell Proliferation
- Infertility and reproductive problems
- Depression
- Dementia
- Endocrine disruption
- Growth problems
- Weight gain
- Premature, delayed puberty
- Goiter
- Pancreatic disorders

Most artificial vectors are from viruses or have viral genes in them, and are programed to cross species barriers and invade genomes. They have the potential to recombine with the genetic material of other viruses to generate new infectious viruses that cross species barriers.

The antibiotic resistance genes carried by artificial vectors can also spread to bacterial pathogens. There is evidence that horizontal gene transfer and recombination have been responsible for creating new viral and bacterial pathogens and for spreading drug and antibiotic resistance among the pathogens.

One way that new viral pathogens may be created is through recombination with dormant, inactive or inactivated viral genetic material that is in all genomes, plants and animals. Recombination between external and resident, dormant viruses have been implicated in many animal cancers.

The cells of all species including our own can take up foreign genetic material. Artificial constructs designed to invade genomes may well invade our own. These insertions may lead to inappropriate inactivation or activation of genes some of which may lead to cancer. Studies reported that as early as 2000, virtually all the seed corn in the U.S. was contaminated with at least a trace of genetically engineered material. Even the organic lots are showing traces of biotech varieties. Controlling the spread of GE contamination is now impossible.

Monsanto's GMO Corn Cause Cancer in rats

Rats are often studied to find out if something is going to be toxic in humans. For the study, some groups of rats got Monsanto's genetically modified roundup-resistant corn. Some got a regular diet but were given water with Roundup in it only a tiny amount that we've been told is safe for us to drink.

Those animals that ate the GMO corn got tumors and died. And the ones that drank the water with roundup in it got tumors and died. The ones that got both developed even more tumors and died. Up to 70 percent of those that got the contaminated water and the genetically modified corn died significantly earlier than the other animals. They developed 2 to 3 times more large cancers than the animals that got no GMO corn or polluted water.   (*see the rats shown on the cover*)

Have you heard of the DARK Act, it stands for Deny Americans the Right to Know whether your food has been genetically engineered. Quaker Oats is one of the largest food companies spending millions of dollars lobbying against the GMO labeling.

The World Health Organization finally labeled the main herbicide used on GMO crops as a probable cause of cancer. GMO crops have led to huge increases in herbicide use, which increases many health issues to our health and untold damage to the environment..

 Monsanto's genetically engineered crops and pesticides they produce are forever changing our world to something of a horror movie. The food you ate as a child is not the same food you are eating today. There are reams of research that shows the link to these GMO Franken foods and the damage to our DNA and the increase of DNA diseases.

It saddens me to say that money is at the root of this soon to be irreversible course that we are unwillingly forced to partake. We are intentionally being lied too and, our elected official are being bought by the highest payer to turn a blind eye.

We are part of a huge experiment that will forever change the course of nature with countless innocent victims. We are perhaps one generation away from irreversible DNA damage. Our children and grandchildren will not be as healthy as we are. Their immune system will be overwhelmed and disease will be the new norm.

Are Genes Transferred alone?

Genes are never transferred alone. Each gene is accompanied by a special piece of genetic material, the promoter, which signals the cell to turn the gene on and transfer the DNA gene sequence into RNA. At the end of the gene there is a terminator signal, to end the transcription and to mark the RNA, so it can be further processed and translated into protein.

The CaMV 35S promoter in transgenic constructs can reactivate dormant viruses or generate new viruses by recombination. The CaMV 35S promoter has been joined artificially to copies of a wide range of viral genomes, and infectious viruses produced in the laboratory. Viral DNA fed to mice is found to reach white blood cells, spleen and liver cells via the intestinal wall, to become incorporated into the mouse cell genome. When fed to pregnant mice, the viral DNA lodged into the cells of the fetuses and the new born animals by crossing the placenta.

Genetically engineered foods are unsafe and the GE food producers do not know where the new genetic material will end up in our food. Food companies are not sure if the new genetic material will destabilize a safe food and make it hazardous. When a GMO is added to our food, our once safe food could become toxic.

The FDA was and is aware of the genetic instability problem prior to establishing their no-testing policy. FDA scientists warned that this problem could create dangerous toxins in food and was a significant health risk to us. The scientists specifically warned that the genetic engineering of foods could result in increased levels of naturally occurring toxins, new toxins, and the increased capability of concentrating toxic substances from the environment (e.g., pesticides or heavy metals).
The FDA scientists recommended that long term toxicological tests be required prior to the marketing of GE foods. FDA officials also were aware that safety testing on the first genetically engineered food, the Calgene Flavr Savr tomato, had shown that consumption of this product resulted in stomach lesions in laboratory rats.

The FDA chose to ignored the toxicity problem with genetically engineered foods. They disregarded their own scientists, undeniable scientific evidence and the deaths and illnesses already attributed to this problem. The FDA refused to require pre-market toxicology testing for GE foods or any toxicity monitoring. The FDA made these decisions with no scientific basis and without public input or independent scientific review. The FDA's intentional response exposes us to harm, yet ensuring profits to corporations.

What about Allergic Reactions?

The genetic engineering of food creates two s serious health risks involving allergies. Genetic engineering can transfer allergens from foods which we know causes allergies, to foods we think are safe.

A study by the New England Journal of Medicine reported that, when a gene from a Brazil nut was engineered into soybeans, people allergic to nuts had serious reactions from the engineered soybeans.

We have no way of avoiding potentially serious health consequences of eating GE foods containing hidden allergenic material. Genetic engineered foods are creating many different and new allergic responses. Each GE food contains new proteins in the form of altered genes, bacteria, viruses, promoters, marker systems, and vectors, which have never been part of our diet.

These new proteins are creating allergic response in some people. The FDA is aware of this new and potentially massive allergy problem. Scientists repeatedly warned that genetic engineering could produce a new protein allergen. FDA officials ignored their own scientists' concerns over the antibiotic resistance genes in human food.

Another hidden risk of GE foods is that they could make disease-causing bacteria resistant to current antibiotics, resulting in an increase in the spread of infections and diseases in the human population.

Virtually all genetically engineered foods contain antibiotic resistance markers which help the producers identify whether the new genetic material has actually been transferred into the host food. The insertion of antibiotic marker genes into our food supply, has weakened antibiotics all but useless in fighting human diseases.

A genetically engineered corn plant from Novartis includes an ampicillin-resistance gene. Ampicillin is an antibiotic used to treat infections in humans and animals. Some European countries refused to permit the Novartis Bt corn to be grown, because of health concerns that the ampicillin resistance gene could move from the corn into bacteria in the food chain, making ampicillin in-effective in fighting bacterial infections.

The risk to human health from antibiotic resistance developing in microorganisms is one of the major public health threats that we are now facing.

The British medical journal, The Lancet, published an important study conducted by Drs. Arpad Pusztai and Stanley W.B. Ewen.

The scientists found that the rats consuming genetically altered potatoes

showed significant detrimental effects on organ development, body metabolism, and immune function.
The biotechnology industry launched a major attack on Dr. Pusztai and his study. Twenty-two leading scientists declared that animal test results linking genetically engineered foods to immuno-suppression are valid.

Genetic engineering can also alter the nutritional value of food. The FDA's Divisions of Food Chemistry & Technology and Food Contaminants Chemistry examined the problem of nutrient loss in GE foods.
The scientists warned the FDA that the genetic engineering of foods could result in undesirable alteration in the level of nutrients in our foods. The FDA ignored findings by their own scientists and never required the foods to mandatory government testing of any sort.

Do corporations have mandates to make a profit at our expense?
Yes, publicly traded corporations do have a legal mandate to pursue a profit, regardless of the harm caused to us. Corporations now control our government and our society.
Corporations are self-governing and they dictate to the government and influence policies that govern our everyday life. No one person is in control and no one person is responsible. This is the advantage of corporations and the danger, especially if the goal is to increase profits.
In 1886 the Supreme Court declared that corporations should be protected by the fourteenth Amendment. The fourteenth Amendment was passed for the protection of freed slaves, which guarantees the Rights to due process of the law and equal protection of the laws.
In 1934 President Franklin D Roosevelt created the New Deal. The New Deal was hated by many business leaders and a small group of them plotted to overthrow Roosevelt's administration. The goal of the New Deal was to curb the control of corporations and help everyday people make a living.

When Ronald Reagan became president he gutted the New Deal. Corporations could now dictate the economic policies of the government. Ronald Reagan removed laws, which protected workers, the environment, reduce taxes, and stripped social programs with no concern for the harm caused to us.

What is the Best interest of the corporation's principle?
Corporate managers and directors have a legal duty to put shareholders' interest above all others and no legal authority to serve any other interest. This has become known as the best interests of the corporation's principle. The law forbids any other motivation for their actions, whether to assist workers, improve the environment, or help consumers save money. corporate social responsibility is illegal.

Some American companies made large profits by working for Adolf Hitler during World War Two. Adam Opel AG, a German automobile maker owned and controlled by General Motors built trucks for the German Army, aircraft parts, and engines for the German fighter bombers. Wladawsky-Berger IBM's vice president of technology helped Hitler with the Nazi extermination and slave labor programs. IBM provided the Nazi with Hollerith tabulation machines used in concentration camps. IBM technicians maintained the machines, IBM engineers trained the users and IBM supplied the punch cards for the machines.

Corporations influence our political processes; to ensure that the government does not restrict their freedoms and slow their profit goals. They spend millions of dollars each year to a political environment that promotes their bottom line and help them survive. The mangers have no authority, to act out of concern for society or to avoid causing harm to people and the environment.

Chapter 2

BABY FOODS WITH GENETICALLY ENGINEERED INGREDIENTS

Milk and soy protein is the foundation used in most infant formulas and these products are often comes from cows injected with rbGH. Many brands also add GE-derived corn syrup or corn syrup solids.

Nestle Infant Formulas
• Carnation Baby Cereals with Formula
• Carnation Baby Formula
• AlSoy
• Good Start
• Follow-Up
• Follow-Up Soy

Nabisco (Phillip Morris)
• Arrowroot Teething Biscuits
• Infant formula Carnation Infant Formulas(Nestle)
• AlSoy
• Good Start
• Follow-Up
• Follow-Up Soy

Enfamil Infant Formulas
(Mead Johnson)
• Enfamil with Iron
• Enfamil Low Iron
• Enfamil A.R.
• Enfamil Nutramigen
• Enfamil Lacto Free
• Enfamil 22
• Enfamil Next step (soy & milk-based varieties)
• Enfamil Pro-Soybee

Isomil Infant Formulas (Abbot Labs)
• Isomil Soy
• Isomil Soy for Diarrhea
• Similac(Abbot Labs)
• Similac Lactose Free

- Similac with Iron
- Similac Low Iron
- Similac Alimentum

Bread with Genetically Engineered Ingredients

Holsum (Interstate Bakeries)
- Holsum Thin Sliced
- Roman Meal
- 12 Grain
- Round Top
- Home Pride
- Buttertop White
- Buttertop Wheat

Pepperidge Farms (Campbell's)
- Cinnamon Swirl
- Light Oatmeal
- Light Wheat
- 100% Whole Wheat
- Hearty Slices
- 7 Grain
- 9 Grain
- Crunchy Oat
- Whole Wheat
- Light Side
- Oatmeal
- Wheat
- 7 Grain
- Soft Dinner Rolls
- Club Rolls
- Sandwich Buns
- Hoagie Rolls

Thomas' (Bestfoods)
- English Muffins Original
- Cinnamon Raisin
- Honey Wheat
- Oat Bran
- Blueberry
- Maple French Toast
- Toast-r-Cakes Blueberry
- Toast-r-Cakes Corn Muffins

Wonder (Interstate Bakeries)
• White Sandwich Bread
• Country Grain
• Buttermilk
• Thin Sandwich
• Light Wheat
• 100% Stoneground Wheat
• Fat Free Multigrain
• Premium Potato
• Beefsteak Rye
• Wonder Hamburger Buns

Potassium Bromate (aka bromated flour)
is made from the toxic chemical bromine. It is used to reduce baking time,
strengthen dough and add bulk to flour. Bromine is a poisonous chemical,
which is known to cause gastrointestinal discomfort, nervous system
disorders and kidney disorders. California states if Potassium Bromate is
used in food products a warning label has to be placed on the food item.
Some countries have banned the use of Potassium Bromate; China, Europe
and Canada.

Breakfast foods with Genetically Engineered Ingredients

Kellogg's
• Pop Tarts (all varieties)
• Pop Tarts Snack Stix (all)
• Nutri-Grain Bars (all)
• Nutri-Grain Fruit Filled Squares (all)
• Nutri-Grain Twists (all)
• Fruit-Full Squares (all)

Nabisco (Nabisco/Phillip Morris)
• Fruit & Grain Bars (all varieties)
• Nature Valley (General Mills)
• Oats & Honey Granola Bars
• Peanut Butter Granola Bars
• Cinnamon Granola Bars

Pillsbury (General Mills)
 Toaster Scrambles & Strudels (all varieties)
Quaker

- Chewy Granola Bars (all varieties)
- Fruit & Oatmeal Bars (all varieties)
- Aunt Jemima Frozen Waffles
- Buttermilk
- Blueberry

Eggo Frozen Waffles (Kellogg's)
- Homestyle
- Buttermilk
- Nutri-Grain Whole Wheat
- Nutri-Grain Multi Grain
- Cinnamon Toast
- Blueberry
- Strawberry
- Apple Cinnamon
- Banana Bread

Hungry Jack Frozen Waffles (Pillsbury/General Mills)
- Homestyle
- Buttermilk

Cereal with Genetically Engineered Ingredients

General Mills
- Cheerios
- Wheaties
- Total
- Corn Chex
- Wheat Chex
- Lucky Charms
- Trix
- Kix
- Golden Grahams
- Cinnamon Grahams
- Count Chocula
- Honey Nut Chex
- Frosted Cheerios
- Apple Cinnamon Cheerios
- Multi-Grain Cheerios
- Frosted Wheaties
- Brown Sugar & Oat Total
- Basic 4
- Reeses Puffs

- French Toast Crunch

Kellogg's
- Frosted Flakes
- Corn Flakes
- Special K
- Raisin Bran
- Rice Krispies
- Corn Pops
- Product 19
- Smacks
- Froot Loops
- Marshmallow Blasted Fruit Loops
- Apple Jacks
- Crispix
- Smart Start
- All-Bran
- Complete Wheat Bran
- Complete Oat Bran
- Just Right Fruit & Nut
- Honey Crunch Corn Flakes
- Raisin Bran Crunch
- Cracklin' Oat Bran

Country Inn Specialties (all varieties)
- Mothers Cereals (Quaker)
- Toasted Oat Bran
- Peanut Butter Bumpers
- Groovy Grahams
- Harvest Oat Flakes
- Harvest Oat Flakes w/Apples & Almonds
- Honey Round Ups

Post (Kraft-Phillip Morris)
- Raisin Bran
- Bran Flakes
- Grape Nut Flakes
- Grape Nut O's
- Fruit & Fibre date, raisin and walnut
- Fruit & Fibre peach, raisin and almond
- Honey Bunch of Oats
- Honey Nut Shredded Wheat
- Honey Comb
- Golden Crisp

- Waffle Crisp
- Cocoa Pebbles
- Cinna-Crunch Pebbles
- Fruity Pebbles
- Alpha-Bits
- Post Selects Cranberry Almond
- Post Selects Banana Nut Crunch
- Post Selects Blueberry Morning
- Post Selects Great Grains

Quaker
- Life
- Cinnamon Life
- 100% Natural Granola
- Toasted Oatmeal
- Toasted Oatmeal Honey Nut
- Oat Bran
- Cap'n Crunch
- Cap'n Crunch Peanut Butter Crunch
- Cap'n Crunch Crunchling Berries

Chocolate with Genetically Engineered Ingredients

Cadbury (Cadbury/Hershey's)
- Mounds
- Almond Joy
- York Peppermint Patty
- Dairy Milk
- Roast Almond
- Fruit & Nut
- Hershey's
- Kit-Kat
- Reese's Peanut Butter Cups
- Mr. Goodbar
- Special Dark
- Milk Chocolate
- Kisses
- Symphony

Kraft (Kraft/Phillip Morris)
- Toblerone (all varieties)
- Mars

- M&M (all varieties)
- Snickers
- Three Musketeers
- Milky Way
- Twix

- Nestle
- Crunch
- Milk Chocolate
- Chunky
- Butterfinger
- 100 Grand

Carnation (Nestle)

Hot Cocoa Mixes:
- Rich Chocolate
- Double Chocolate
- Milk Chocolate
- Marshmallow Madness
- Mini Marshmallow
- No Sugar

Hershey's
- Chocolate Syrup
- Special Dark Chocolate Syrup
- Strawberry Syrup

Nestle
- Nesquik
- Strawberry Nesquik

Swiss Miss (ConAgra)
- Chocolate Sensation
- Milk Chocolate
- Marshmallow Lovers
- Marshmallow Lovers Fat Free
- No Sugar Added

Chapter 3
Condiments with Genetically Engineered Ingredients

Del Monte (Nabisco/Phillip Morris)
• Ketchup
• Heinz
• Ketchup (regular & no salt)
• Chili Sauce
• Cocktail Sauce
• Heinz 57 Steak Sauce

Hellman's (Bestfoods)
• Real Mayonnaise
• Light Mayonnaise
• Low-Fat Mayonnaise

• Hunt's (ConAgra)
• Ketchup (regular & no salt)
• KC Masterpiece
• Original BBQ sauce
• Garlic & Herb Marinade
• Honey Teriyaki Marinade

Kraft (Kraft/Phillip Morris)
• Miracle Whip (all varieties)
• Kraft Mayonnaise (all)
• Thick & Spicy BBQ sauces (all varieties)
• Char Grill BBQ sauce
• Honey Hickory BBQ sauce

Nabisco (Nabiso/Phillip Morris)
• A-1 Steak Sauce
• Open Pit (Vlasic/Campbells)
• BBQ sauces (all)
• Chi-Chi's (Hormel)
• Fiesta Salsa (all varieties)
• Old El Paso (Pillsbury)
• Thick & Chunky Salsa
• Garden Pepper Salsa
• Taco Sauce
• Picante Sauce

Ortega (Nestle)
• Taco Sauce
• Salsa Prima Homestyle
• Salsa Prima Roasted Garlic
• Salsa Prima 3 Bell Pepper
• Thick & Chunky Salsa

Pace (Campbells)
• Chunky Salsa
• Picante Sauce

Tostitos Salsa (Frito-Lay/Pepsi)
• All Natural
• All Natural Thick & Chunky
• Roasted Garlic
• Restaurant Style

Cookies with Genetically Engineered Ingredients

Delicious Brands (Parmalat)
• Animal Crackers
• Ginger Snaps
• Fig Bars
• Oatmeal
• Sugar-Free Duplex
• Honey Grahams
• Cinnamon Grahams
• Fat Free Vanilla Wafers
• English Toffee Heath Cookies
• Butterfinger Cookies
• Skippy Peanut Butter Cookies

Famous Amos (Keebler/Flowers Industries)
• Chocolate Chip
• Oatmeal Raisin
• Chocolate Sandwich
• Peanut Butter Sandwich
• Vanilla Sandwich
• Oatmeal Macaroon Sandwich

Frookies (Delicious Brands/Parmalat)
• Peanut Butter Chunk

- Chocolate Chip
- Double Chocolate
- Frookwich Vanilla
- Frookwich Chocolate
- Frookwich Peanut Butter
- Frookwich Lemon
- Funky Monkeys Chocolate
- Ginger Snaps
- Lemon Wafers

Keebler (Keebler/Flowers Industries)
- Chips Deluxe
- Sandies
- E.L. Fudge
- Soft Batch Chocolate Chip
- Golden Vanilla Wafers
- Droxies
- Vienna Fingers
- Fudge Shoppe Fudge Stripes
- Fudge Shoppe Double Fudge & Caramel
- Fudge Shoppe Fudge Stix
- Fudge Shoppe Peanut Butter Fudge Stix
- Country Style Oatmeal
- Graham Originals
- Graham Cinnamon Crisp
- Graham Chocolate
- Graham Honey Low Fat
- Crème Filled Wafers
- Chocolate Filled Wafers

Nabisco (Nabisco/Phillip Morris)
- Oreo,(all varieties)
- Chips Ahoy!(all varieties)
- Fig Newtons (and all Newtons varities)
- Lorna Doone
- Nutter Butters
- Barnum Animal Crackers
- Nilla Wafers
- Nilla Chocolate Wafers
- Pecanz Shortbread
- Family Favorites Oatmeal
- Famous Wafers
- Fudge Covered Mystic Sticks

- Honey Maid Graham Crackers
- Honey Maid Cinnamon Grahams
- Honey Maid Chocolate Grahams
- Honey Maid Oatmeal Crunch
- Teddy Grahams
- Teddy Grahams Cinnamon
- Teddy Grahams Chocolate
- Teddy Grahams Chocolate Chips
- Café Cremes Vanilla
- Café Crème Cappuccino

Pepperidge Farm (Campbell's)
- Milano
- Mint Milano
- Chessmen
- Bordeaux
- Brussels
- Geneva
- Chocolate Chip
- Lemon Nut
- Shortbread
- Sugar
- Ginger Men
- Raspberry Chantilly
- Strawberry Verona
- Chocolate Mocha Salzburg
- Chocolate Chunk Chesapeake
- Chocolate Chunk Nantucket
- Chocolate Chunk Sausalito
- Oatmeal Raisin Soft Baked

Sesame Street (Keebler)
- Cookie Monster
- Chocolate Chip
- Chocolate Sandwich
- Vanilla Sandwich
- Cookie Pals
- Honey Grahams
- Cinnamon Grahams
- Frosted Grahams

- Snack Wells (Nabisco/Phillip Morris)
- Devil's Food

- Golden Devil's Food
- Mint Crème
- Coconut Crème
- Chocolate Sandwich
- Chocolate Chip
- Peanut Butter Chip
- Double Chocolate Chip

Chapter 4
Crackers with Genetically Engineered Ingredients

Keebler (Keebler/Flowers Industries)
• Town House
• Club
• Munch 'Ems (all varieties)
• Wheatables
• Zesta Saltines
• Toasteds (Wheat, Onion, Sesame & Butter Crisps)
• Snax Stix (Wheat, Cheddar & original)
• Harvest Bakery (Multigrain, Butter, Corn Bread)

Nabisco (Nabisco/Phillip Morris)
• Ritz (all varieties)
• Wheat Thins (all)
• Wheatsworth
• Triscuits
• Waverly
• Sociables
• Better Cheddars
• Premium Saltines (all)
• Ritz Snack Mix (all)
• Vegetable Flavor Crisps
• Swiss Cheese Flavor Crisps
• Cheese Nips (all)
• Uneeda Biscuits

Pepperidge Farm (Campbell's)
• Butter Thins
• Hearty Wheat
• Cracker Trio
• Cracker Quartet
• Three Cheese Snack Stix
• Sesame Snack Stix
• Pumpernickel Snack Stix
• Goldfish (original, cheddar, parmesan, pizza, pretzel)
• Goldfish Snack Mix (all)

Red Oval Farms (Nabisco/Phillip Morris)

- Stoned Wheat Thin (all varieties)
- Crisp N Light Sourdough Rye
- Crisp N Light Wheat

Sunshine (Flowers Industries)
- Cheeze-It (original & reduced fat)
- Cheeze-It White Cheddar
- Cheeze-It Party Mix
- Krispy Original Saltines

Frozen Dinners with Genetically Engineered Ingredients

Banquet (ConAgra)
- Pot Pies (all varieties)
- Fried Chicken
- Salisbury Steak
- Chicken Nugget Meal
- Pepperoni Pizza Meal

Budget Gourmet (Heinz)
- Roast Beef Supreme
- Beef Stroganoff
- Three Cheese Lasagne
- Chicken Oriental & Vegeatble
- Fettuccini Primavera

Green Giant (Pillsbury)
- Rice Pilaf with Chicken Flavored Sauce
- Rice Medley with Beef Flavored Sauce
- Primavera Pasta
- Pasta Accents Creamy Cheddar
- Create-a-Meals Parmesan Herb Chicken
- Cheesy Pasta and Vegetable
- Beef Noodle
- Sweet & Sour
- Mushroom Wine Chicken

Healthy Choice (ConAgra)
- Stuffed Pasta Shells
- Chicken Parmagiana
- Country Breaded Chicken
- Roast Chicken Breast
- Beef Pot Roast

- Chicken & Corn Bread
- Cheese & Chicken Tortellini
- Lemon Pepper Fish
- Shrimp & Vegetable
- Macaroni & Cheese

Kid Cuisine (ConAgra)
- Chicken Nugget Meal
- Fried Chicken
- Taco Roll Up
- Corn Dog
- Cheese Pizza
- Fish Stix
- Macaroni & Cheese

Lean Cuisine (Stouffer's/Nestle)
- Skillet Sensations Chicken & Vegetable
- Broccoli & Beef
- Homestyle Beef
- Teriyaki Chicken
- Chicken Alfredo
- Garlic Chicken
- Roast Turkey

Hearty Portions Chicken Florentine
- Beef Stroganoff
- Cheese & Spinach Manicotti
- Salisbury Steak

Café Classics Baked Fish
- Baked Chicken
- Chicken a L'Orange
- Chicken Parmesan
- Meatloaf with Whipped Potatoes

Everyday Favorites Chicken Fettuccini
- Chicken Pie
- Angel Hair Pasta
- Three Bean Chili with Rice
- Macaroni & Cheese

Marie Callenders (ConAgra)
- Chicken Pot Pie

- Lasagna & Meat Sauce
- Turkey & Gravy
- Meat Loaf & Gravy
- Country Fried Chicken & Gravy
- Fettuccini with Broccoli & Cheddar
- Roast Beef with Mashed Potatoes
- Country Fried Pork Chop with Gravy
- Chicken Cordon Bleu

Ore-Ida Frozen Potatoes (Heinz)
- Fast Fries
- Steak fries
- Zesties
- Shoestrings
- Hash Browns
- Tater Tots
- Potato Wedges
- Crispy Crunchies

Rosetto Frozen Pasta (Heinz)
- Cheese Ravioli
- Beef Ravioli
- Italian Sausage Ravioli
- Eight Cheese Stuffed Shells
- Eight Cheese Broccoli Stuffed Shells

Stouffer's (Nestle)
- Family Style Favorites Macaroni & Cheese
- Stuffed Peppers
- Broccoli au Gratin
- Meat Loaf in Gravy
- Green Bean & Mushroom Casserole

- Homestyle Meatloaf
- Salisbury Steak
- Chicken Breast in Gravy

- Hearty Portions Salisbury Steak
- Chicken Fettucini
- Meatloaf with Mashed Potatoes
- Chicken Pot Pie

Swanson (Vlasic/Campbells)

- Meat Loaf
- Fish & Chips
- Salisbury Steak
- Chicken Nuggets
- Hungry Man Fried Chicken
- Roast Chicken
- Fisherman's Platter
- Pork Rib

Voila! (Bird's Eye/Agri-Link Foods)
- Chicken Voila! Alfredo
- Chicken Voila! Garlic
- Chicken Voila! Pesto
- Chicken Voila! Three Cheese
- Steak Voila! Beef Sirloin
- Shrimp Voila! Garlic

Weight Watchers (Heinz)
- Smart Ones Fiesta Chicken
- Basil Chicken
- Ravioli Florentine
- Fajita Chicken
- Roasted Vegetable Primavera

Heat & Serve Meals with Genetically Engineered Ingredients

Chef Boyardee (ConAgra)
• Beefaroni
• Macaroni & Cheese
• Mini Ravioli
• ABC's & 123's

Dinty Moore (Hormel)
• Beef Stew
• Turkey Stew
• Chicken & Dumplings
• Hormel
• Chili with Beans
• Chili No Beans
• Vegetarian Chili with Beans

Kids' Kitchen (Hormel)
• Spaghetti Rings with Meatballs
• Macaroni & Cheese
• Pizza Wedges with 3 Cheese

Franco-American (Campbell's)
• Spaghetti O's
• Mini Ravioli
• Power Rangers Pasta in Sauce

Meat & Dairy Alternatives with Genetically Engineered Ingredients

Loma Linda(Worthington/Kellogg's*)
• Meatless Chik Nuggest

Morningstar (Worthington/Kellogg's*)
• Harvest Burger
• Better 'n Burgers
• Garden Veggie Patties
• Grillers Burgers
• Black Bean Burger
• Chicken Patties

Natural Touch (Worthington/Kellogg's*)
• Garden Vegetable Pattie
• Black Bean Burger
• Okra Pattie
• Lentil Rice Loaf
• Nine Bean Loaf

Worthington (Worthington/Kellogg's*)
• Vegetarian Burger
• Savory Slices

Dairy Alternatives

Nutra Blend Soy Beverage(Bestfoods)
• Original
• Vanilla
• Apple
• Orange
*A company letter states that they are in the process of converting to non-genetically modified "proteins" in all products.

Meal Mixes & Sauce Packets with Genetically Engineered Ingredients

Betty Crocker (General Mills)
• Garden Vegetable Pilaf
• Creamy Herb Risotto
• Garlic Alfredo Fettuccini
• Bowl Appetit Cheddar Broccoli
• Macaroni & Cheese
• Pasta Alfredo
Knorr (Bestfoods)
• Mushroom Risotto Italian Rice
• Broccoli au Gratin Risotto
• Vegetable Primavera Risotto
• Risotto Milanese
• Original Pilf
• Chicken Pilaf
• Rotini with 4 Cheese
• Bow Tie Pasta with Chicken & Vegetable
• Penne with Sun-Dried Tomato
• Fettuccini with Alfredo
• Classic Sauce Packets Hollandaise

Béarnaise
- White
- Brown
- Lemon Herb
- Mushroom Brown
- Onion
- Roasted Chicken
- Roasted Pork
- Roasted Turkey

Pasta Sauce Packets Alfredo
- Four Cheese
- Carbonara
- Pesto
- Garlic Herb

Lipton (Unilever)
- Rice & Sauce Packets Chicken Broccoli
- Cheddar Broccoli
- Beef Flavor
- Spanish
- Chicken Flavor
- Creamy Chicken
- Mushroom

Sizzle & Stir Skillet Supers Lemon Garlic Chicken & Rice
- Spanish Chicken & Rice
- Herb Chicken & Bowties
- Cheddar Chicken & Shells

Near East (Quaker)
- Spicy Tomato Pasta Mix
- Roasted Garlic & Olive Oil Pasta Mix
- Falafel Mix
- Lentil Pilaf
- Couscous
- Tomato Lentil
- Parmesan
- Toasted Pinenut
- Herb Chicken
- Broccoli & Cheese
- Curry

• Pasta Roni (Quaker)
• Fettuccini Alfredo
• Garlic Alfredo
• Angel Hair Pasta with Herbs
• Angel Hair Pasta with Parmesan Cheese
• Angel Hair Pasta with Tomato Parmesan
• Angel Hair Pasta Primavera
• Garlic & Olive Oil with Vermicelli

Rice-a-Roni (Quaker)
• Rice Pilaf
• Beef
• Chicken
• Fried Rice
• Chicken & Broccoli
• Long Grain & Wild Rice
• Broccoli au Gratin

Uncle Ben's (Mars)
• Long Grain & Wild Rice (Original & with Garlic)
• Brown & Wild Rice Mushroom
• Country Inn Mexican Fiesta
• Country Inn Oriental Fried Rice
• Country Inn Chicken & Vegetable
• Country Inn Chicken & Broccoli
• Natural Select Chicken & Herb
• Natural Select Tomato & Basil
• Chef's Recipe Chicken & Vegetable Pilaf
• Chef's Recipe Beans & Rice
• Chef's Recipe Broccoli Rice

Frozen Pizza with Genetically Engineered Ingredients

Celeste (Aurora Foods)
• Supreme
• Pepperoni
• Vegetable
• Four Cheese
• Deluxe
• Cheese

Tombstone (Kraft/Phillip Morris)
• Pepperoni
 •Supreme
• Sausage & Pepperoni
• Extra Cheese
• Stuffed Crust
• Three Cheese

Totino's (Pillsbury)
• Crisp Crust
• Pepperoni
• Combination

Chapter 5

SALAD DRESSING WITH GENETICALLY ENGINEERED INGREDIENTS

Hellman's (Unilever/Bestfoods)
• Creamy Ranch
• Blue Cheese
• Italian
• Fat Free Ranch
• Fat Free Italian
• Citrus Splash (all varieties)

Hidden Valley (Clorox)
• Original Ranch
• Light Ranch
• French Onion Ranch
• Sour Cream Ranch
• BLT Ranch
• Italian Herb & Cheese
• Ranch with Bacon
• Honey & Bacon French

Kraft Dressings (Kraft/Phillip Morris)
• Thousand Island
• Ranch
• Roka Blue Cheese
• Zesty Italian
• Creamy Parmesan Romano
• Seven Seas Creamy Russian
• Seven Seas Italian
• Seven Seas Viva Italian
• Seven Seas Red Wine Vinegar
• Fat Free Ranch
• Fat Free Blue Cheese
• Fat Free French
• Fat Free Honey Dijon
• Caesar Parmesan Vinaigrette
• Roasted Garlic Vinaigrette

Marie's (Dean Foods)
- Parmesan Ranch
- Chunky Blue Cheese
- Tangy French
- Thousand Island
- Parmesan Ranch
- Chunky Feta Cheese
- Pourable Ranch
- Pourable Italian
- Pourable Thousand Island
- Pourable Caesar
- Fat Free Blue Cheese
- Fat Free Raspberry Vinaigrette
- Fat Free Italian Vinaigrette
- Fat Free Red Wine Vinaigrette
- Fat Free Honey Dijon Vinaigrette

Wishbone Dressings (Lipton/Unilever)
- Ranch
- Chunky Blue Cheese
- Olive Oil Vinaigrette
- Sun-Dried Tomato Vinaigrette
- Caesar Parmesan Vinaigrette
- Roasted Garlic Vinaigrette
- Fat Free Wine Vinaigrette
- Deluxe French
- Oriental
- Just 2 Good Italian
- Just 2 Good Country Italian
- Just 2 Good Parmesan Basil

Snack Foods with Genetically Engineered Ingredients

Act II Microwave Popcorn (ConAgra)
• Butter
• Extreme Butter
• Corn on the Cob

Frito-Lay* (PepsiCo)
• Lays Potato Chips (all varieties)
• Ruffles Potato Chips (all)
• Doritos Corn Chips (all)
• Tostitos Corn Chips (all)
• Fritos Corn Chips (all)
• Cheetos (all)
• Rold Gold Pretzels (all)
• Cracker Jack Popcorn

Healthy Choice Microwave Popcorn (ConAgra)
• Organic Corn (soy/canola oils)

Mothers Corn Cakes (Quaker)
• Butter Pop

Orville Redenbacher Microwave Popcorn (ConAgra)
• Original
• Homestyle
• Butter
• Smart Pop
• Pour Over
• Orville Redenbacher Popcorn Cakes
• Chocolate
• Caramel
• Orville Redenbacher Mini Popcorn Cakes
• Butter
• Peanut Caramel
• Chocolate Peanut

Pop Secret Microwave Popcorn (Betty Crocker/General Mills)
• Natural
• Homestyle
• Jumbo Pop

- Extra Butter
- Light
- 94% Fat Free Butter

Pringles (Procter & Gamble)
- Original
- Low Fat
- Pizza-licious
- Sour Cream & Onion
- Salt & Vinegar
- Cheezeums
- Quaker Rice Cakes
- Peanut Butter
- Chocolate Crunch
- Cinnamon Streusel
- Mini
- Chocolate
- Ranch
- Sour Cream & Onion
- Apple Cinnamon
- Caramel Corn
- Quaker Corn Cakes
- White Cheddar
- Caramel Corn
- Strawberry Crunch
- Caramel Chocolate Chip

*Frito has informed its corn and potato suppliers that the company wishes to avoid GE crops, but acknowledges that canola or other oils and ingredients in its products may be from GE sources.

Soda & Juice Drinks with Genetically Engineered Ingredients
Coca Cola (Coca Cola)
- Sprite
- Cherry Coke
- Barq's Root Beer
- Minute Maid Orange
- Minute Maid Grape
- Surge
- Ultra
- PepsiCo
- Pepsi
- Slice
- Wild Cherry Pepsi

- Mug Root Beer
- Mountain Dew
- Cadbury/Schweppes
- 7-Up
- Dr. Pepper
- A & W Root Beer
- Sunkist Orange
- Schweppes Ginger Ale

Capri Sun juices (Kraft/Phillip Morris)
- Red Berry
- Surfer Cooler
- Splash Cooler
- Wild Cherry
- Strawberry Kiwi
- Fruit Punch
- Pacific Cooler
- Strawberry
- Orange
- Grape

Fruitopia (Coca Cola)
- Grape Beyond
- Berry Lemonade
- Fruit Integration
- Kiwiberry Ruckus
- Strawberry Passion
- Tremendously Tangerine

Fruit Works (PepsiCo)
- Strawberry Melon
- Peach Papaya
- Pink Lemonade
- Apple Raspberry

Gatorade (Quaker)
- Lemon Lime
- Orange
- Fruitpunch
- Fierce Grape
- Frost Riptide Rush

Hawaiian Punch (Procter & Gamble)
• Tropical Fruit
 •Grape Geyser

Chapter 6
Energy Bars & Drinks with Genetically Engineered Ingredients

Power Bars
Power Bar (Nestle)
• Oatmeal Raisin
• Apple Cinnamon
• Peanut Butter
• Vanilla Crisp
• Chocolate Peanut Butter
• Mocha
• Banana
• Wild Berry
• Harvest Bars Apple Crisp
• Blueberry
• Chocolate Fudge Brownie
• Strawberry
• Peanut Butter Chocolate Chip

Drink Mixes

Carnation Instant Breakfast Mix (Nestle)
• Creamy Milk Chocolate
• Classic Chocolate
• French Vanilla
• Strawberry
• Café Mocha

Soup with Genetically Engineered Ingredients

Campbell's
• Tomato
• Chicken Noodle
• Cream of Chicken
• Cream of Mushroom
• Cream of Celery
• Cream of Broccoli
• Cheddar Cheese
• Green Pea
• Healthy Request Chicken Noodle
• Cream of Chicken

- Cream of Mushroom
- Cream of Celery
- Campbell's Select Roasted Chicken with Rice

- Grilled Chicken with Sundried Tomatoes
- Chicken Rice
- Vegetable Beef

- Chunky Beef with Rice
- Hearty Chicken & Vegetable
- Pepper Steak
- Baked Potato with Steak & Cheese
- New England Clam Chowder

Soup to Go Chicken Noodle
- Chicken Rice
- Garden Vegetable
- Vegetable Beef & Rice

Simply Home Chicken Noodle
- Chicken Rice
- Garden Vegetable
- Vegetable Beef with Pasta

Healthy Choice (ConAgra)
- Country Vegetable
- Fiesta Chicken
- Bean & Pasta
- Chicken Noodle
- Chicken with Rice
- Minestrone

Pepperidge Farms (Campbell's)
- Corn Chowder
- Lobster Bisque
- Chicken & Wild Rice
- New England Clam Chowder
- Crab Soup

Progresso (Pillsbury)
- Tomato Basil
- Chicken Noodle
- Chicken & Wild Rice

- Chicken Barley
- Lentil
- New England Clam Chowder
- Zesty Herb Tomato
- Roasted Chicken with Rotini
- Fat Free Minestrone
- Fat Free Chicken Noodle
- Fat Free Lentil
- Fat Free Roast Chicken

Chapter 7

Frozen Pizza with Genetically Engineered Ingredients

Celeste (Aurora Foods)
• Supreme
• Pepperoni
• Vegetable
• Four Cheese
• Deluxe
• Cheese

Tombstone (Kraft/Phillip Morris)
• Pepperoni
• Supreme

Tomatoes & Sauces with Genetically Engineered Ingredients
Del Monte (Nabisco/Phillip Morris)
• Tomato Sauce

Five Brothers Pasta Sauces (Lipton/Unilever)
• Summer Vegetable
• Five Cheese
• Roasted Garlic & Onion
• Tomato & Basil

Healthy Choice Pasta Sauces (ConAgra)
• Traditional
• Garlic & Herb
• Sun-Dried Tomato & Herb

Hunts (ConAgra)
• Traditional Spaghetti Sauce
• Four Cheese Spaghetti Sauce
• Tomato Sauce
• Tomato Paste

Prego Pasta Sauces (Campbells)
• Tomato, Basil & Garlic
• Fresh Mushroom
• Ricotta Parmesan

- Meat Flavored
- Roasted Garlic & Herb
- Three Cheese
- Mini-Meatball
- Chicken with Parmesan

Ragu Sauces (Lipton/Unilever)
- Old World Traditional
- Old World with Meat
- Old World Marinara
- Old World with Mushrooms
- Ragu Robusto Parmesan & Romano
- Ragu Robusto Roasted Garlic
- Ragu Robusto Sweet Italian Sausage
- Ragu Robusto Six Cheese
- Ragu Robusto Tomato, Olive Oil & Garlic
- Ragu Robusto Classic Italian Meat
- Chunky Garden Style Super Garlic
- Chunky Garden Style Garden Combo
- Chunky Garden Style Tomato, Garlic & Onion
- Chunky Garden Style Tomato, Basil & Italian Cheese
- Pizza Quick Traditional

Chapter 8

Soda & Juice Drinks with Genetically Engineered Ingredients

Coca Cola (Coca Cola)
- Sprite
- Cherry Coke
- Barq's Root Beer
- Minute Maid Orange
- Minute Maid Grape
- Surge
- Ultra
- PepsiCo
- Pepsi
- Slice
- Wild Cherry Pepsi
- Mug Root Beer
- Mountain Dew

- Cadbury/Schweppes
- 7-Up
- Dr. Pepper
- A & W Root Beer
- Sunkist Orange
- Schweppes Ginger Ale

Capri Sun juices (Kraft/Phillip Morris)
- Red Berry
- Surfer Cooler
- Splash Cooler
- Wild Cherry
- Strawberry Kiwi
- Fruit Punch
- Pacific Cooler
- Strawberry
- Orange
- Grape

Fruitopia (Coca Cola)
- Grape Beyond
- Berry Lemonade
- Fruit Integration

- Kiwiberry Ruckus
- Strawberry Passion
- Tremendously Tangerine

Fruit Works (PepsiCo)
- Strawberry Melon
- Peach Papaya
- Pink Lemonade
- Apple Raspberry

Gatorade (Quaker)
- Lemon Lime
- Orange
- Fruitpunch
- Fierce Grape
- Frost Riptide Rush

Hawaiian Punch (Procter & Gamble)
- Tropical Fruit
- Grape Geyser

Hi-C (Coca Cola)
- Pink Lemonade
- Watermelon Rapids
- Boppin' Berry
- Tropical Punch
- Smashin' Wildberry
- Blue Cooler
- Blue Moon Berry
- Orange
- Cherry

Kool Aid (Kraft/Phillip Morris)
- Blastin' Berry Cherry
- Bluemoon Berry
- Kickin' Kiwi Lime
- Tropical Punch
- Wild Berry Tea
- Ocean Spray
- Cranberry Juice Cocktail
- Cranapple
- CranGrape
- CranRaspberry

- CranStrawberry
- CranMango

Squeeze It (Betty Crocker/General Mills)
- Rockin' Red Puncher
- Chucklin' Cherry
- Mystery 2000

Sunny Delight (Procter & Gamble)
- Sunny Delight Original
- Sunny Delight With Calcium Citrus Punch
- Sunny Delight California Style Citrus Punch
- Tang juices (Kraft/Phillip Morris)
- Orange Uproar
- Fruit Frenzy
- Berry Panic

Tropicana Twisters (PepsiCo)
- Grape Berry
- Apple Raspberry Blackberry
- Cherry Berry
- Cranberry Raspberry Strawberry
- Pink Grapefruit
- Tropical Strawberry
- Orange Cranberry
- Orange Strawberry Banana

V-8 (Campbells)
- V8 Tomato Juices (all varieties)
- Strawberry Kiwi
- Strawberry Banana
- Fruit Medley
- Berry Blend
- Citrus Blend
- Apple Medley
- Tropical Blend
- Island Blend

Brominated vegetable oil
Brominated vegetable oil also known as BVO, interferes with our body's' iodine receptors sites and cause bromated thyroid or bromism. Brominated vegetable oil causes thyroid diseases i.e., hypothyroidism, hyperthyroidism,

thyroid cancer, and autoimmune disease.

BVO has been linked to schizophrenia, birth defects, hearing loss, and growth problems. Bromine competes with iodine in our bodies for absorption. The more bromine we consume, the less iodine is available for the thyroid gland to produce thyroid hormone. Hence our bodies need iodine to make thyroid hormone.

Brominated vegetable oil has a bromine molecule attached to it. Bromine is a poisonous chemical that is corrosive and toxic; it is band in more than 100 countries. In the United States, it is permitted in food and soft drinks i.e., Mountain Dew, Crush Orange, Sundrop, Squirt, Gatorade Orange, Crush Peach, Crush Pineapple, Strawberry Powerade, Fanta, Dr. Pepper, Fresca, Sunkist Orange, and others.

When bromine is added to vegetable oil, it makes the vegetable oil viscosity the same as water, so the flavoring stays mixed in the soft drink and they don't separate. Brominated vegetable oil is found in more than 10% of soft drinks in the United States.

Chapter 9

CAMPBELL'S SOUP WITH GENETICALLY ENGINEERED INGREDIENTS

- Tomato
- Chicken Noodle
- Cream of Chicken
- Cream of Mushroom
- Cream of Celery
- Cream of Broccoli
- Cheddar Cheese
- Green Pea
- Healthy Request
- Chicken Noodle
- Cream of Chicken
- Cream of Mushroom
- Cream of Celery
- Campbell's Select
- Roasted Chicken with Rice
- Grilled Chicken with Sundried Tomatoes
- Chicken Rice
- Vegetable Beef
- Chunky
- Beef with Rice
- Hearty Chicken & Vegetable
- Pepper Steak
- Baked Potato with Steak & Cheese
- New England Clam Chowder
- Soup to Go
- Chicken Noodle
- Chicken Rice
- Garden Vegetable
- Vegetable Beef & Rice
- Simply Home
- Chicken Noodle
- Chicken Rice
- Garden Vegetable
- Vegetable Beef with Pasta

Healthy Choice (ConAgra)
- Country Vegetable
- Fiesta Chicken

- Bean & Pasta
- Chicken Noodle
- Chicken with Rice
- Minestrone

Pepperidge Farms (Campbell's)
- Corn Chowder
- Lobster Bisque
- Chicken & Wild Rice
- New England Clam Chowder
- Crab Soup

Progresso (Pillsbury)
- Tomato Basil
- Chicken Noodle
- Chicken & Wild Rice
- Chicken Barley
- Lentil
- New England Clam Chowder
- Zesty Herb Tomato
- Roasted Chicken with Rotini
- Fat Free Minestrone
- Fat Free Chicken Noodle
- Fat Free Lentil
- Fat Free Roast Chicken

TOMATOES & TOMATOES SAUCES WITH GENETICALLY ENGINEERED INGRIDENTS
(Nabisco/Phillip Morris)

- Tomato Sauce

Pasta Sauces Five Brothers (Lipton/Unilever)
- Summer Vegetable
- Five Cheese
- Roasted Garlic & Onion
- Tomato & Basil

Healthy Choice Pasta Sauces (ConAgra)
- Traditional
- Garlic & Herb
- Sun-Dried Tomato & Herb

Hunts(ConAgra)
- Traditional Spaghetti Sauce
- Four Cheese Spaghetti Sauce

- Tomato Sauce
- Tomato Paste
- Summer Vegetable
- Five Cheese
- Roasted Garlic & Onion
- Tomato & Basil

Healthy Choice Pasta Sauces (ConAgra)
- Traditional
- Garlic & Herb
- Sun-Dried Tomato & Herb

Hunts(ConAgra)
- Traditional Spaghetti Sauce
- Four Cheese Spaghetti Sauce
- Tomato Sauce
- Tomato Paste

Prego Pasta Sauces (Campbells)
- Tomato, Basil & Garlic
- Fresh Mushroom
- Ricotta Parmesan
- Meat Flavored
- Roasted Garlic & Herb
- Three Cheese
- Mini-Meatball
- Chicken with Parmesan

Ragu Sauces (Lipton/Unilever)
- Old World Traditional
- Old World with Meat
- Old World Marinara
- Old World with Mushrooms
- Ragu Robusto Parmesan & Romano
- Ragu Robusto Roasted Garlic
- Ragu Robusto Sweet Italian Sausage
- Ragu Robusto Six Cheese
- Ragu Robusto Tomato, Olive Oil & Garlic
- Ragu Robusto Classic Italian Meat
- Chunky Garden Style Super Garlic
- Chunky Garden Style Garden Combo
- Chunky Garden Style Tomato, Garlic & Onion
- Chunky Garden Style Tomato, Basil & Italian Cheese
- Pizza Quick Traditional

Chapter 10
Monosodium Glutamate- What is Monosodium Glutamate?

According to the FDA, Monosodium Glutamate is a food additive that can be added to any food in any amount. Vegetarian foods are a favorite place to hide MSG.

The History of Monosodium Glutamate

During World War II, Japanese soldier's military rations tasted better than rations from other militaries. This was a great interest to the U.S. military and many food processing companies. In 1948 representatives Of the U.S. military, Oscar Mayer, General Foods, Campbell and many other companies in the food industries meet at a symposium in Chicago.

The Japanese secret ingredient Monosodium Glutamate was unveiled. MSG made canned and frozen food taste as good as homemade food and kids would crave more.

Does MSG kill Brain Cells?

Monosodium Glutamate, passes quickly into the blood stream and enters the brain and other organs directly. MSG causes the neurons to (nerve ending in the brain and others organs) to fire uncontrollably. The brain translates this overstimulation of the nerves into what we believe to be delicious taste and scrumptious flavor.

Two to twenty-four hours later, the entire neuron and its synapses are dead. Our brain cells are constructed to last our entire lifetime. In a few short hours, monosodium glutamate has excited many of our brain cells to death.

When MSG is injected under the skin of newborn mice and rats, it causes the rodents to grow obese beyond their normal range. When MSG is injected directly into a subjects brain cells, it quickly and completely kills them dead.

Mice and rats are tested with experimental drugs meant of humans, because their physiology closely mimics humans. When mice are treated with MSG they experience hyperinsulinemia, a condition where the pancreas excretes huge amounts of insulin.

What are the Side effects of MSG?

Asthma, behavioral problems, stomach cramps, chest discomforts, headaches, stomach aches, tiredness, depression, Nausea, dizziness, loss of bladder/bowel control, rage reactions, and hostility to other children.

What does the FDA know about MSG?

The FDA is aware that Monosodium Glutamate in foods is not as safe as they claim. The FDA reported that between 1980 and 1994, there were 622 reports of complaints about side effects from MSG. Research show overwhelming and undeniable evidence the eating MSG can do long term, irreversible damage to the body.

What happens to your Fetus when exposed to MSG?

When a developing fetus is exposed to high levels of monosodium glutamate in the mothers diet, it could make the infant more prone to weight gain later in life.

Not only can exposure to MSG predispose children to obesity, but it can reduce their activity level and hinder their ability to lose excess weight even though they eat less than other children.

The expectant mother's diet can be consumed by the fetus growing inside of her through the umbilical cord and the placenta. The placenta acts as a barrier to regulate the flow of amino acids to the fetus.

Researchers have found that not only do amino acids and toxins cross the barrier to the baby, but they tend to collect there so the concentration are higher in the growing fetus than in the mother's blood.

MSG In Low Fat Foods

Even after we eat low fat, low calorie foods, the level of insulin rises in the blood. The MSG in the low fat, low calorie foods stimulates our pancreas, to release fat-creating insulin. The insulin searches for any sugar it can turn into adipose tissue and store it as fat.

Fat molecules give most of the flavor in our food. Diet foods have the fat removed, but monosodium glutamate is added. The FDA has no limit to how much glutamate can be add.

When MSG causes increased insulin, we lose the motivation to exercise. The hyperinsulinemia sends large amounts of insulin to remove almost all the blood sugar it can find. Low blood sugar leaves us feeling drained and tired.

Research showed that (MSG) monosodium glutamate lowers the amount of growth hormone present during the development stage. Females subjects respond to MSG induced obesity in far more extreme way than males.

What about MSG and Diabetes?

Diabetes is the number one cause of death by disease in North America. Diabetes is the leading cause of blindness, it increases the chance of heart disease, it accounts for more than a quarter of all new cases of kidney disease, and it is the reason of 50% of limb amputations throughout the world.

Diabetes occurs when the pancreas is unable to produce enough insulin to regulate the sugar levels in the blood. High doses of monosodium glutamate produce hyperinsulinemia, where the pancreas abnormally increases the amount of insulin in the blood.
When the pancreas pumps out more than normal amount of insulin it continues to function. But the increased work load can be too much and the pancreas fails with the end result of Diabetes.

The effects MSG on the Pancreas

Our Pancreas regulates sugar (glucose) levels in the blood. When the sugar level in the blood is high, the Beta Cells within the Pancreas produce insulin. Monosodium Glutamate in the blood stream can bypass control of the Pancreas and hyper stimulate the beta-cells to over produce insulin.
The over production of insulin is called Hyperinsulinemia leading to obesity. Hyperinsulinemia facilitates sugar (glucose) storage as fat, which can be the first step in diabetes. The pancreas being over stimulated by monosodium glutamate starts to malfunction.
Meanwhile Beta – Cells start deteriorating and the body's T-cell immune response will shut them down. As the pancreas malfunctions a little more each day, it can be maintained functional by pills and diet until it can no longer produce enough insulin.
Eventually the pills are exchanged for insulin injections. Monosodium glutamate stimulates the Beta-Cells of the pancreas to death, leaving a life sentence of diabetes.

MSG & the Eyes:

Our eyes are extremely sensitive to changes in Glutamate levels. The capillaries in the eyes easily transport glutamate directly into the sensitive areas of the eye. Researchers found that a diet of monosodium glutamate over period years could result in retinal cell destruction and total blindness.

Glutamate in the eyes latches onto glial cells which support vision and excites them to death. When ingesting large amounts of MSG in their diets, diabetics could increase their chances of going blind.

MSG & Blood Brain Barrier:

Researchers have shown that MSG crosses the Blood Brain Barrier. The FDA states the MSG cannot cross the Blood Brain Barrier. The Ajinomoto Company (MSG manufacturer) Website, states that L-Glutamate (MSG) and ammonia can pass through the blood brain barrier.

The FDA has overlooked the fact that the blood brain barrier is not infallible and can fail in many situations. Increased physical stress of a short duration can increase the ease with which larger molecules can cross into the brain.

Brain injury (stroke or trauma), where a blood vessel breaks and bleed into the brain, allows direct access for the monosodium glutamate to cross the barrier and enter the brain.

Allergies create an increase of histamines in the blood. Histamines dilate the arterioles, allowing for larger molecules to enter the brain.

The hypothalamus is a brain organ that regulates hormones throughout the body linked to growth and the control of the pituitary gland. The Hypothalamus does not have a blood barrier, and is affected by MSG in the blood stream. The lack of protection from glutamates can allow monosodium glutamate to impair memory and damage neurons in the hypothalamus.

MSG, Headaches, and Migraines.

MSG has been established as a trigger for headaches. Even the FDA admits that headaches are a side effect of eating MSG. High Glutamate content within the spinal cord can also induce headaches. Both chronic tension headaches and chronic daily headaches can be linked to Glutamate.

Headaches and migraines in children have been linked to Monosodium Glutamate in their diet. Research has shown that 100% of people who ate

MSG laced foods and then fasted overnight complained of headaches. When large amounts of MSG gather within the developing fetus, the increased state of Glutamate excitotoxicty could alter the brain itself in the developing stage. Neuronal pathways growing in the developing brain could be excited into greater, more rapid development.

The brain could be over-stimulated so that some areas could become hyper-sensitized to Glutamate, while other areas could be overdeveloped to the point of cellular death. ADHD infants show susceptibility to high levels of Glutamates within their neuronal regions.

MSG & Autism

Autism is an ailment that manifest as the retardation of the mental abilities of the individuals. Children with this disorder can have extreme anti-social behaviors, act abusive to others or themselves, practice repetitive motion; show delayed and reduced language development and use, as well as other socially unacceptable behaviors.

Autism develops in the fetus during pregnancy and occurs more often within the same family. Males make up 75% of individuals with Autism and females 25%. The research reports on autism notes that individuals with the disorder have extreme Glutamate level abnormalities and Glutamate receptors anomalies within the brain.

The brain's speech area (Brocca) and other sensitive cells could be stimulated to death, therefore those parts of the brain maybe totally unusable. This damage could explain the brain abnormalities seen in people with autism. Family genetics may decide how much monosodium glutamate it takes to affect the developing fetus brain.

MSG & Schizophrenia

Schizophrenia disorder exhibits signs of brain dysfunction from hallucinations to episodes of mania. Research shows that the common link between people with schizophrenia is an imbalance of brain chemistry, notably a defect involving the glutamatergic system.

The brain of people with this disorder are unable able to process glutamate in the same way unaffected people brain does. The reduced ability of the brain to transmit glutamate results in the disturbed information process that is seen in the schizophrenic population.

MSG's ability to kill receptive brain cells could lead to a debilitating reduction in gluamatergic receptor cells in the brain. Therefore the schizophrenic's brain cannot process glutamate transmissions properly. Alterations in glutamate receptors of the schizophrenic brain have been observed in studies.

MSG & Epilepsy

Epilepsy is a misfiring of the brains nerves which causes seizures. Monosodium glutamate is used to create epileptic seizures in animal's studies when scientists want to induce epileptic seizures.

Monosodium L-Glutamate (MSG) a commonly used food additive induces convulsive disorders in rats. Epilepsy affects 1% of the population and affects children and the elderly more often than any other population.
MSG is not needed by our bodies and it has no nutritional value. MSG is put in food for two reasons and to make us eat more of that food which means more profit for the food manufactures. MSG in one form or another has found its way into almost every processed food.

Chapter 11
What are the dangers of milk?

The dangers of milk are allergies, asthma, behavioral problems, cancer, diabetes, digestive problems, and many more health problems for human consumers.

History of dairy Cows in America
Cows are not indigenous to this country. Imagine what the Native Americas thought when they saw those first cows being unloaded from the pilgrim ship Charity. In 1624 a bull and three cows where imported to Plymouth Massachusetts.
Pilgrim's used cow's milk for butter. There was no way to store milk, so it was made into butter. Most cows where only able to produce 1 quart per day. The early cows in this country where able to roam free and eat grass all day long. Native Americans received their first taste dairy from the pilgrims.

What makes Cow's Milk Unhealthy?

Cow's milk is now unhealthy for human consumption. It often comes from diseased cows that are harbingers of dangerous and disease-causing substances that have disastrous effect in the human body.

Cows' milk also has cholesterol, fat, and 59 active hormones. When we and our children drink that cold glass of liquid protein, we also drink pus, blood, feces, growth hormones, cholesterol, pesticides, added vitamin D-3, bacteria, viruses, bovine leukemia, bovine tuberculosis, and bovine immunodeficiency virus.
Calcium
We were told as children, if we drink milk we would get calcium for strong bones and teeth. Cows get calcium for their bones from plants. Plants have large amounts of magnesium which is necessary for the body to absorb and utilize the calcium.
Research shows that nations with the highest amount of dairy consumption also have the highest rates of osteoporosis. Calcium from cow milk is deficient in magnesium, which is needed for calcium absorption and use in the human body.

Vitamin D-3 and CROHN'S DISEASE

Vitamin D-3 always is derived from four different animal sources. Pig skin, pig brains, sheep skin, and raw fish liver. Most of the time, Vitamin D-3 is extracted from pig skin and sold to dairy processors.

Johne's disease is caused by Mycobacterium Para tuberculosis. Cows diagnosed with Johne's disease have diarrhea, and heavy fecal passing of bacteria. The bacteria are not destroyed by pasteurization. The milk-borne bacteria begin to grow in the human stomach and cause irritable bowel syndrome and Crohn's Disease.

Mad Cow Disease and Pesticides

There may also be prions (pronounced PREons) in the milk and meat. Prions are crystalline substances that act like a virus with no DNA or RNA. Prions it can incubate for a period of 5 to 30 years, finally ending in Mad Cow Disease.

A 2004 study by the FDA resulted in the following findings of pesticides in Milk.

• Ninety-six percent of samples contained DDT, which was banned from agricultural use in the early 1970s.

• Nearly 99 percent contained diphenylamine (DPA), an industrial chemical used for many purposes in manufacturing rubber and plastic parts, and in making certain drugs.

• Forty-one percent of samples contained dieldrin, a banned organochlorine pesticide. Endosulfan sulfate, an endocrine disrupter, found in numerous toxicological studies to pose serious developmental risks during pregnancy and to infants and children as their bodies grow and mature, turned up in 18 percent of samples.

• About a quarter of samples had synthetic pyrethroid insecticides. Nearly 9 percent of samples contained, 3-hydroxycarbofuran, a highly-toxic breakdown product of the carbamate insecticide.

Antibiotics in Milk

The FDA requires each truck-load of milk to be tested for 4 antibiotics. Two of the four are amoxicillin and ampicillin, but there are more than 20 that are not tested for. When the dairy cows have exceeded their usefulness, they are taken to the slaughterhouse for slaughtering.

The meats from these cows have high levels of antibiotics and end up on our plates. Federal inspectors find illegal antibiotics in hundreds of older dairy cows marked for the slaughterhouse.

The Wall Street Journal (Dec. 1989) did a study of the antibiotic residues in milk on the market and found that 20% had illegal antibiotics present. This was confirmed in May 1992 in a Consumers Reports study and the Center for Science in the Public Interest found 38% contained illegal antibiotics.

What's in a Cows' diets?

Cows' diets are now supplemented with bone meal, blood meal, and ground body parts from (recycled protein) slaughter houses. Sometimes roasted chicken feces are added for extra protein. Cows are now injected with genetically modified bovine growth hormones. These new hormones allow the dairy cows to produce greater amount of milk.

Genetically modified Bovine growth Hormones

All milk has naturally occurring growth hormones which is for the baby calf to start growth. Those natural occurring hormones have been genetically modified and combined with the genetic material from bacteria. When a hormone is recombined with the genetic material from another species of animal, the new hormone has "r" placed before it.

Five errors were created when producing the Posilac (rbGH) shot. The report by (Richard, Odaglia & Deslex, 1989) has been hidden from the public under former President Bill Clinton's Trade Secrets act.

rGBH causes an 80% increase in IGF-1 which is a powerful growth hormone found in all milk in low quantities. The elevated levels of IGF-1 can fuel cancer to grow at a high rate, or cause cancer cells that would have been destroyed by the body's immune system to proliferate. IGF-1 is a key factor in the rapid growth and proliferation of breast, prostate and colon cancers, and likely it promotes all cancers.

On November 5, 1993 the FDA approved the use of a genetically engineered recombinant bovine growth hormone. The natural growth hormone was taken from the dairy cows and recombined with the genetic material of bacteria, then implanted inside of E. coli bacteria. The resulting bacteria produce large amounts of bovine growth hormones.

The public does not know if they are drinking milk that has been treated with genetically recombined hormone and recombined with E. coli bacteria. The rBGH injections cause continuous increases of IGF-1 Insulin-like Growth Factor-levels. IGF-1 occurs naturally in human beings as well as cows.

IGF-1 is not destroyed by pasteurization; it survives the digestion process, is absorbed into the blood, and produces potent growth promoting effects. This portion of the report to the FDA was covered up as a trade secret. IGF-1 helps transform normal breast tissue to cancerous cells, and enables malignant human breast cells to invade and spread to distant organs.

Increases risk of infections- and Drug use in Dairy Cows
Posilac (trade name for rBGH) produced by Monsanto, has an insert in the package warning of the increased risk of mastitis (an infection of the udder), a painful infection in the breast tissue of a lactating mammal.

Mastitis is treated with antibiotics; sometimes it's not treated at all. If not treated it results in high amounts of white blood cells and secretions (pus). An increase of almost 80% infection rate in rBGH-treated herds means farmers have to treat their cows with more drugs, as stated on the drug package insert.

I can go on and on with documentation supporting the deliberate misuse of our food supply in the name of greed. We are paying a high cost for this greed by companies and the support from the government agencies that are supposed to protect us.

Chapter 12
Dangers of Fluoride

Fluoride is toxic and dangerous to the human body. It's amazing and sad how the supporters hid the overwhelming evidence of the harmful effect this poison has on the human body. Politics and greed seem to be the overwhelming influence to prevent the truth from being published.

History shows blatant and intentional lies to cover up the damage that is done to us and our children. This is not a comprehensive review of its' dangers to the human body, but some of the worst case scenarios.

Researcher at Harvard School of Dental Medicine Cover Up

Chester Douglass, a researcher at Harvard School of Dental Medicine misrepresented the results of an unpublished study about bone cancer and fluoridated tap water, indicating there was no increased risk of bone cancer. Soon it was discovered that Douglass had suppressed the data and was ignoring the fact that bone cancer could result, especially in children. In 2006 the actual facts were published and showed a fivefold increased risk for a rare type of bone cancer in boys.

The government assigned the project to a National Academy of Sciences expert panel for review. However vested interest groups gained control of the panel membership and lobbied forcefully to limit what the panel could actually study, this was done to prevent a financial ruin.

The panel was prevented from evaluating the 0.7 to 1.2 range and was instructed to only evaluate the 4 mg/L upper range of safety. Therefore any adverse panel findings would only relate to naturally occurring toxic levels, and not to the ADA recommended level of fluoride added to water.

On March 22, 2006, the National Academy of Sciences (NAS) released their review of fluoride, in the context of 4 mg/L as the safe upper limit of exposure. The panel concluded that, the EPA standard of 4mg/L does not protect against adverse health effects. People drinking water at those levels over their lifetime has increased risk for bone fractures.

Fluorosis

Fluorosis is the abnormal effect that fluoride has on the formation of tooth enamel. This means that exposure may interfere with the normal development of the structural integrity of tooth enamel. This results in visible tooth discoloration and can lead to brown marks on the teeth, and with more advanced cases, severe staining, enamel loss, and pitting or mottling of teeth.

Dentists have been and are well aware of these adverse effects. However they justify it by saying that the benefits of cavity reduction are more important than the discoloration of teeth. They support an opinion that brown teeth are a cosmetic issue, not a health issue.

The National Academy of Sciences countered this opinion. They stated children consuming 4mg/L of fluoride "are at risk of developing severe tooth enamel fluorosis, a condition that can cause tooth enamel loss and pitting." They also redefined fluorosis as a health condition, not a cosmetic problem.

The majority of the members (10 of 12) judged the condition to be an adverse health effect enamel loss and pitting can compromise the ability of the tooth enamel to protect the dentin and ultimately, the pulp from decay and infection.

The National Academy of Science report also details the harmful effects on bone metabolism, since fluoride accumulates in bone over the course of a lifetime. In bone, fluoride acts to promote abnormal bone-cell growth.
This gives the appearance of improved bone density, but it's creating abnormal bone growth that results in weak bones, increased risk for fractures and possibility of bone cancer. These effects are likely to be greatest in children, because it becomes built into their bones during high-growth phase.

The National Academy of Science report also details how thyroid hormone function is disrupted and is common in America. Up until the 1970's European physicians used low doses of fluoride to suppress the function of the thyroid gland as a treatment for hyperthyroidism.

Bone Toxin

The truth is that fluoride is a powerful bone toxin, drawn into the bone and teeth, especially during growth, where it acts to weaken the bone and to weaken the teeth. The panel also stated further research for risks involving endocrine effects and brain function and the suggested that certain individuals be evaluated for psychological, behavioral, or social effects.

The federal government and many local governments are actively administering this harmful poison to over 200 million Americans. What right does a government have to force poison on us? Furthermore the government has failed to warn citizens that this poison may cause osteoporosis and cancer.

The FDA knows that sodium fluoride is toxic. They have even banned it from being added to food. According to the FDA it is illegal for a company to add even a drop in food you eat, but is added to water we drink.

EPA public stance on Fluoride

The EPA public stance on water fluoridation is to promote it. However the workers within the EPA have another view. The National Treasury Employees Union Local 2050 represents 1500 scientist, lawyers, engineers and other professional employees at the EPA headquarters in Washington.
The union took the stand that not only is water fluoridation poisonous, but it should be immediately terminated.
A document titled Why EPA Headquarters' Union of Scientist Opposes Fluoridation, date May 1st, 1999, and prepared on behalf of the Union Chapter Senior Vice President, J. William Hirzy, outlines the EPA employees stands with absolute clarity.

The Union document states that the employees at the EPA headquarters in Washington supported the value of water fluoridation until 1985, when one of their scientists was pressured by management to make a false statement supporting the safety of fluoridation in water if the limits were raised to 4mg/Liter 4ppm. It was reported that the increased of allowable levels was demanded of the EPA by political forces.

The demand by management for an EPA scientist to support fraudulent statements raised concern within the employees at the EPA. They started researching the side effects of fluoride in water.

The EPA Headquarters employees union made the following startling discoveries:
• Human's brain and kidneys are being damaged with 1part per million

dosages they currently get in the water supply.

• Can cause neurotoxic effects like hyperactivity.

• Lead to a drop of 5-10 IQ points in children.

• Reduce the pineal gland's ability to produce the hormone Melatonin: thereby disturbing sleep patterns and also quickening the onset of puberty in children.

• Increase the occurrence of the cancer Osteosarcoma.

• Causes skeletal fluorosis, leading to an increase of incidence of bone fractures in communities with this water treatment.

• Applied in toothpaste and gels can cause gene mutations and cancerous tumor growth.

The EPA employees were very alarmed by these findings. The friction between the union and management became more heated when Dr. William Marcus, Chief Toxicologist of the Office of Drinking Water was fired from the EPA for refusing to remain silent about the cancer risks of water fluoridation.

The employees of the government recognized the dangers of, but the administration at the EPA and the U.S. Public Health Service promotes it.

Mind-control drug, during World War 11
ALCO, the world largest producer of aluminum (owned by the Mellon family), has a long and sordid corporate history. ALCO's mission was formed during the era of Rocker feller ethics. ALCO signed contracts with the Nazis to supply aluminum to Germany prior to World War 11, instead of to America, which gave the enemy a military advantage. Contracts with IG Farben enabled Bayer to become one of the largest producers in the world.

During World War 11, the Russians and the Nazis used fluoride to make their prisoners dispirited and controllable because it was an excellent mind-control drug.
Tooth Paste and Fluoride
Sodium Fluoride used for water came from aluminum smelting (still use in tooth paste). Two different forms are now used in our water supply: silica fluoride and sodium fluorosilicate. People now receive it from many other

sources besides water.
Other sources include

• food and beverages processed with fluoridated water
• dental treatments
• mechanically deboned meat
• tea
• Pesticide residues (e.g., from cryolite) on food.
• It is now broadly acknowledged that exposure to non-water sources has significantly increased since the water fluoridation program first began.

No disease has ever been linked to a fluoride deficiency, nor has a single biological process has been shown to require it. However there is extensive evidence that it can affect many important biological processes and interfere with numerous enzymes.

Chapter 13
Escherichia coli, E. coli O157:H7

The bacteria Escherichia coli were named for the Austrian doctor, Theodor von Escherich (1857-1911), who first isolated the bacteria belonging to the family enterobacteriaceae, Eschericheae. E.coli bacteria aid the breakdown of cellulose and assists in the absorption of vitamin K.

E. coli O157:H7, which was first identified in 1982, is a deadly version of E.coli
E. coli O157:H7 is a mutant form of E.coli, found in the intestinal tract of cattle .
• E coli 0157: H7 can release two powerful toxins called Verotoxin or a Shiga toxin.
• The Verotoxin binds to receptors on the human kidney, brain and intestinal cells and kills them.
• Shiga toxins can attack the lining of the intestines.

Infected Cattle Meat

According the United States Department of Agriculture, the meat from cattle, is sterile. It is only after this meat comes in contact with the contents of the intestines or the feces of infected cattle does it become contaminated.
The pathogens from infected cattle are spread in feedlots, slaughter houses, and hamburger grinders. The slaughter house contamination of meat can occur during removal of animal hides and removal of digestive systems.

If the hides are not properly cleaned, dirt and manure can fall into the meat. When stomachs and intestines are pulled out of cattle, if not done correctly the contents of the digestive system can spill everywhere. Widespread contamination is higher when the meat is processed into ground beef.
The pathogens from infected cattle are spread in feedlots;
• Were cattle may defecate
• Urinate onto each other.
• Their hides are covered with filth before they are slaughtered where it takes only a very small amount of contamination to infect the meat.

• Sometimes the animal carcass falls unto the filthy floor of the slaughter house and it is hung back on the line with insufficient or no cleaning.
• Sometimes during the cutting of the carcass, the intestines of the animal are accidentally sliced and their contents explode over the exposed meat.

Meat inspection laws

The meat inspection laws of this country where passed in 1907. These laws only allowed the government meat inspectors to perform limited inadequate testing of meat. Current FDA regulations allow the following to be rendered into cattle feed

• dead pigs
• dead horses
• dead poultry

The regulations not only allow cattle to the fed dead poultry they also allow poultry to be fed dead cattle. Cattle blood is still put into the feed given to American cattle. This is a flagrant disregard of our health.

Hamburger meat

Hamburger meat is the most common meat to be infected with the E. coli O157:H7 bacteria. This is because the hamburgers we eat contain meat from up to 100 different head of cattle. Usually they are not the finest top quality animals that are ground up as hamburger, but old non-milk producing cows.

This is especially true of hamburger meat fed to our children in school lunch programs. It only takes a microscopic amount Escherichia coli, E. coliO157:H7 in meat from one infected animal to contaminate an entire batch of meat. Finally, this large batch of meat is divided and sent to stores and restaurants throughout a large geographic area.

Through DNA testing it was determined that the Jack-in-the-Box hamburger meat contained Escherichia coli, E. coli O157:H7 which killed six year-old Lauren Rudolph from Carlsbad, CA in December 1992, was the same Jack-in-the-Box hamburger meat which killed people in the State of Washington as well as Las Vegas, NV in January and February 1993.

McDonald's hamburgers in Canada

In 1977 there was an outbreak of E. coli O157:H7 which was traced to McDonald's hamburgers in Alberta, Canada. The symptoms included severe abdominal cramps, followed by bloody diarrhea. Some of the infected people developed hemolytic uremic syndrome (HUS), which shuts down the kidneys and then attacks and shut down other organs in the body. At present, there is no cure for HUS, and it is very often fatal. Hemolytic Uremic Syndrome (HUS) is the leading cause of kidney failure in children. Dr. Mohammed Karmali, a Canadian medical researcher found the correlation between the hamburger meat and Escherichia coli, E. coli O157:H7

After the Jack-in-the-Box outbreak in early 1993, there have been over 100 other outbreaks in this country. The USDA believes that the incidences of E.coli poisoning are increasing.

E. coli O157:H7 primarily affects children and senior citizens. 13 year-old Eric Mueller of Oceanside, CA died in November 1993 after eating a cheeseburger at a local fast food restaurant. 18 year-old Laura Day was stricken after eating a hamburger while attending the University of Alabama shortly before Thanksgiving 1993. Laura spent 42 days in the hospital and her family spent over one-quarter million dollars for her treatment.

Our Kids are at risk when they eat Hamburgers!

Parents our kid's health is at risk! After eating a hamburger at a San Diego Jack in the Box, six year old Lauren Beth Rudolph was admitted to the hospital on Christmas Eve. She suffered from excruciating pain, had three heart attacks, and died on December 28th 1992 in her mother's arms. Test of the hamburgers patties disclosed that presence of E. Coli O157: H7.

In January of 1993, doctors at a hospital in Seattle Washington treated children with bloody diarrhea. Some were suffering from hemolytic uremic syndrome, a disorder that causes kidney damage. Health officials traced the outbreak of food poisoning to undercooked hamburgers at local Jack in the box restaurant.

Internal Damage

In about 4 % of reported E coli 0157: H7 cases, the Shiga toxins enter the bloodstream, causing hemolytic uremic syndrome, which can lead to kidney failure, anemia, internal bleeding, and destruction of the vital organs. The Shiga toxins can cause seizures, neurological damage, and strokes.

About 5% of the kids who develop hemolytic uremic syndrome (HUS) are killed by it. Survivors are often left with permanent disabilities, such as blindness or brain damage. The pathogen is the leading cause of Kidney failure among children in the United States. Antibiotics may further damage our kid's health by killing off the pathogen and prompting a sudden release of its Shiga toxins.

What causes E coli 0157: H7 INFECTIONS?

- Infection can be caused from drinking contaminated water,
- swimming in a contaminated lake,

- Playing in a contaminated water park.
- while playing and crawling on contaminated carpet
- The most common cause of foodborne outbreaks has been from eating undercooked ground beef.

E coli 0157: H7 outbreaks have also been caused by
- contaminated bean sprouts,
- salad greens,
- cantaloupe,
- salami,
- raw milk
- under pasteurized apple cider.

All of those foods most likely had come in contact with cattle manure. The E coli 0157: H7 pathogen may also be spread by the feces of:
- deer
- dogs
- horses
- flies
- Our kid's health is at risk due to exposure to home pets, which have been fed infected cattle.

Weak FDA Regulations

Recent changes in how cattle are raised, slaughtered and processed have created an ideal environment for pathogens to spread. Cattle are packed into feedlots standing in pools of manure with little exercise.

About 75% of the cattle and the United States were routinely fed to livestock wastes, the rendered remains of dead sheep and dead cattle until August of 1997. There were also fed millions of dead cats and dead dogs every year, purchased from animal shelters.

The FDA banned such practices after evidence from Great Britain suggested that they were responsible for widespread outbreak of bovine spongiform encephalopathy also known as mad cow disease.

The waste products from poultry plants, including saw dust and old newspapers used as litter are also fed to cattle. Chicken manure may contain dangerous bacteria such as salmonella and Campylobacter, parasites such as tapeworms and Giardia Lamblia, antibiotics residues, arsenic and heavy metals.

Factory Slaughter Houses

Factory slaughter houses and grinders dominate the nation production of ground beef. The modern processing plant can produce 1000,000 pounds of hamburger a day. A single animal infected with the E coli 0157: H7 can contaminate thousands of pounds of hamburger meat. A large percentage of this meat is served in our schools, placing millions of our kids' health at risk.

Animals used to make about ¼ nation's ground beef are worn out dairy cattle, are animals most likely to be disease and have antibiotics residue. The mixtures of animals in most American ground beef plants play a crucial role in spreading E. coli O157:H7. A fast food hamburger now contains meat from dozens or even hundreds of different cattle.

Most hamburgers are bought at fast food restaurants where our kids, eat more of them than anyone else. Our kids' health is not for sale to the highest special group. It is up to us as parents to look after our children well-being.

Men's Health, Estrogen, Hamburgers, Sperm, and Testosterone

Estrogen is the hormone that makes women feminine. Each man has some estrogen, but when its' not in balance, it can create havoc in your body.
Estrogen promoters
Some estrogen promoters includes
• pesticides
• herbicides in fruits and vegetables,
• hormones in meat and dairy,
• soy and products high in soy isoflavones,
• estrogenic isoflavones (such as in the herb black cohosh),
• plastic derivatives in packed food and water,
• diets high in animal fat
excessive consumption of omega 6 rich oils (such as canola, corn, safflower and soy oils).

Processing increases the concentration of the already existing estrogenic compounds in food. Processed soy products may be more estrogenic than soy beans.

Commercially processed milk or whey protein products may be more estrogenic than regular milk or yogurt, unless they're organic.

Phthalates are some of the most common types of estrogenic chemicals, which are mainly used as plasticizers and industrial detergents. They increase plastic flexibility and are often found in food containers, water bottles, vinyl shower curtains, cosmetics, perfumes, dental material and children's toys. .

Xenoestrogens are Estrogenic chemical form of Estrogen and are found in just about everything we come in contact with. Xenoestrogens mimics estrogen activity in the body and it's almost impossible to avoid these estrogen mimickers. Research shows that xenoestrogens disrupt sexual development and reproductive functions in various living species.

The ongoing assaults of these chemicals affect men's health like excess estrogens, with overwhelming and sometimes devastating consequences. Todays' industries are putting hundreds of chemicals into everyday products that mimic the female hormone estrogen and when they get into your blood, they stick to estrogen receptors in your cells.

Estrogenic chemicals are found in:
• in the air
• car emissions
• detergents
• food
• lotions
• paints,
• nail polishes
• plastics
• soaps
• water

Major sources of estrogen chemicals are petroleum based products, pollutants, pesticides, herbicides, fungicides and plastics. When you eat a hamburger, you're getting a dose of estrogen.

Some large cattle ranchers and poultry farmers inject their cattle and chickens with estrogen to plump them up. These toxic estrogens accumulate in the fatty tissues and breast milk of these animals.

When we eat these animals and drink their milk the accumulated estrogen moves from their tissues to our tissues causing adverse effects in men's bodies.

Many of these estrogenic chemicals are found in rivers and lakes, causing severe damages to wildlife marine species. Changes include a decline in the sperm quality of fish, interference with the sexual development of alligators and turtles and the feminization of male frogs. Researchers found recently that about 40% of the male bass in the Potomac River were producing eggs.

Xenoestrogens are causing devastating effects on men's health, potency and the capacity to reproduce. Sperm counts in men are rapidly declining worldwide, and there's a link to these estrogenic chemicals. Researchers in Edinburgh, Scotland, reported that men born after 1970 have a sperm count 35 percent lower than those born before 1959.

Recent reports of men's health are showing a decline of men's testosterone by 20 percent in only one generation. There's very compelling evidence that we're experiencing a significant drop in male fertility and virility.

Testosterone Levels

When a man's estrogen is balanced, his testosterone gets stronger. When estrogen gets out of control, it causes the testosterone to become overwhelmed. Low Free Testosterone predicts mortality from cardiovascular disease.

A man's testosterone to estrogen level should be at least four parts testosterone to one part estrogen. Testosterone has a positive effect on men's health. It helps prevent internal blood clotting, increases blood flow to the heart, and it gives better endothelial function, and helping blood pressure.

How to enhance Men's Health

Certain compounds found in cruciferous vegetables turn the feminizing estrogen into a healthy version. Crucifers are a group of vegetables including broccoli, Brussels sprouts, cauliflower and cabbage. When you eat a vegetable like broccoli, your body breaks it down into different compounds. One of the compounds is isindole-3-carbinol (I3C), a phytochemical.

Isindole-3-carbinol (I3C), helps switch the feminizing estrogens into neutral or even helpful estrogens such as 2-hydroxyestrone. When (I3C) gets into our instestines, part of it converts into DIM (diindolylmethane), an estrogen neutralizer. Isindole -3-carbinol and DIM help clear your body of excess estrogen.

Estrogen inhibiting compounds in plants (flavonoids and indoles) found in passiflora, chamomile, bee products, citrus fruits, onion, garlic, and cruciferous vegetables (broccoli, cauliflower, brussel sprouts and cabbage). Other beneficial estrogen modulators are omega 3 fatty acids (N-3), derived from flaxseeds, hempseeds and fatty fish help support men's health.

Our Liver

Our liver neutralizes and eliminates toxins including estrogenic substances. We can help our livers detoxify our bodies and promote wellness through diet and supplementation. Green vegetables, beets, carrots and berries are dietary liver aids.

Spices, which can also be taken as supplements, include turmeric, oregano, thyme, rosemary, sage and ginger. Herbs like milk thistle, gotu kola, bacopa, amla berries, shilajit and dandelion root are beneficial to men's health.

Chapter 14
Aspartame

In 1965, a researcher at G.D. Searle, James Schlatter accidentally discovered aspartame NutraSweet, while working to find a cure for stomach ulcers. In 1975 G.D Searle had managed to talk the FDA to allow Aspartame use as an artificial sweetener, but not as a food additive. The research left out scientific studies that prove aspartame caused tumors and epileptic seizures in monkeys.

A 1975 FDA Commissioner Dr. Alexander Schmidt appointed a special task force to examine G. D. Searle and its testing methods regarding aspartame. The task force found G D Searle, to be fraudulent and their research on the safety of aspartame.

FDA Chief Counsel Richard Merrell suggested to the U.S. Attorney general, that a grand jury be setup to investigate G. D. Searle. However G.D. Searle was never brought to trial.

Dr. John Only the same scientists who researched the dangers of MSG along with the FDA managed to bring together a board of inquiry to investigate the toxicity of aspartame. In 1980 the board unanimously voted to reject the use of aspartame until further testing could be done in regards to research indicating that it causes brain tumors.

PRESIDENT RONALD REGAN

In 1981 Ronald Regan was president of the United States and Donald Rumsfeld and G.D. Searle applied for a new application to the FDA to declare Aspartame safe as a food additive. In March, the commissioner of the FDA, Jere Goyan established a 5 member panel of scientist to review the issues outlined by the 1980 Public Board of Inquiry. However, President Ronald Regan had other plans and appointed Arthur Hull Hayes, Jr.as the Commissioner of the FDA.

In July, Hayes ignored all the previous findings and declared Aspartame could be added to food. One year; later, it became legal to add it to soft drinks.

Diet Sodas was the new drink of popularity. It was used extensively to supply the troops in action during the Gulf War. Aspartame, known as NutraSweet has been shown to be toxic and cause many health problems.

Aspartame breaks down into its individual's components, methanol and methanol breaks down into formaldehyde. The formaldehyde collects into the tissues of the bodys' organs, especially the liver. Formaldehyde wraps tightly in the DNA and impairs proper function.

NutraSweet website warns of the dangers of methanol breakdown in the body and producing formaldehyde. Many independent studies state that Aspartame consumption may constitutes a hazard.

The American Academy of Clinical Toxicology states that the methanol derived formaldehyde in the body has been linked to nausea, abdominal pain, blindness, and impairment of the central nervous system. Formaldehyde in drinking water has been proven to create cancerous tumors.

Formaldehyde has been known to cause a Chemical Sensitivity Disorder and is closely linked to Chronic Fatigue Syndrome and Fibromyalgia. Research shows that those who were diagnosed Fibromyalgia managed to completely or almost completely reduces the symptoms by removing MSG and Aspartame from their diet.

Methanol, Formaldehyde and Gulf War Syndrome

NutraSweet breaks down to create higher levels of methanol and formaldehyde which mimics symptoms of methanol or formaldehyde poisoning. Gulf War Syndrome has symptoms similar to formaldehyde and methanol poisoning. Most symptoms of Gulf War Syndrome Illness are similar to Chronic Fatigue syndrome and or Fibromyalgia.

Aspartame is linked by two amino acids (aspartic acid, phenylalanine), and methanol alcohol.

Aspartame, Phenylalanine and Phenylketonuria

Some people do not have the necessary coenzyme (Biopterin) to properly metabolize phenylalanine or it is in very low levels. This genetic disorder is called (PKU) phenylketonuria.

The most vulnerable in our society are children and pregnant women. If left untreated, these symptoms could lead to mental retardation, seizure disorders, and even permanent brain damage. Phenylalanine becomes a brain toxin at higher levels especially during brain development in a child.

Pregnant women who have this condition and ingest aspartame during pregnancy have a 93% chance of their baby becoming mentally retarded and a 72% chance their baby will be born with a substantially smaller brain.

But these symptoms can be avoided if identified in blood screenings at or at the time of birth. Treatment typically includes a strict vegan diet for the entire life as well as drugs to regulate the body's cellular health.

Aspartame, Phenylalanine and brain function

All three of these components are known be toxic to the brain especially the developing brain. Phenylalanine is a commonly found amino acid in many foods and is a natural occurring amino acid.

Phenylalanine will interfere with the brain's ability to insulate nerve fibers and with the connections between nerve cells. When this occurs during brain development, it interferes with the maturation of the brain and prevents a normal functioning brain so the child can't have a normal intellection development and speech development.

Severe mental retardation, behavioral problems, severe brain malformation, and frequent cardiac abnormalities are a complete expression of PKU. Millions of people in this country are a carrier of the gene for PKU; both genes are needed to develop the disease.

Children with PKU should be placed on a diet very low in phenylalanine. When phenylalanine is removed from their diet early they don't become mentally retarded or have seizures. If you don't continue to reduce phenylalanine from their diet into later life they will begin to deteriorate.

An elevated blood level of phenylalanine is harmful even to the brain of adolescents, teenagers or even later in life. Children with high blood levels of phenylalanine complained of difficulty concentrating and had emotional instability.

Pregnant women and metabolism of phenylalanine

Is recommended that during pregnancy the blood phenylalanine level should not exceed 6 mg per deciliter and at 10 mg and above there's serious danger to the developing brain of your un-born child.

A woman's metabolism of phenylalanine is abnormal during her pregnancy. Therefore, she's unable to properly metabolize phenylalanine. So her levels of phenylalanine are higher than normal which can cause damage to the brain of her unborn children.

Millions of women who are pregnant each year are in danger of damaging the brains of their unborn children.

The safety level of aspartame set by the FDA is 50mg per Kg. There are over 5000 products, medicine, and drinks that have aspartame in them. We reach levels more than 150 to 200 mg per kg per day, particularly in small children. A can of diet soda has 10mg, so 5 diet sodas a day is 50mg per day.

Aspartame, phenylalanine, formaldehyde and the Thymus gland

If immune cells of the thymus gland are exposed to formaldehyde for 24 hours there is an increase in death of the thymus gland cells at a dose of 50mg of aspartame. We ingest methanol at 6 times higher than the dose that cause death of the cells in the thymus gland.

The thymus gland is responsible for our immunity soon after birth. Damage to it early in life can cause auto immune disease for the rest of our life. The placenta concentrates phenylalanine in the mother's blood and double the amount in the baby's blood.

All three components of aspartame phenylalanine, Aspartic acid and Methanol can either cause seizures or can precipitate seizures in people who have a history of seizures.

Independent studies show that mice that where prone the seizures had an increase in seizures when exposed to aspartame. The higher the dose of aspartame the more seizures where seen. 78 to 100 % of the mice had seizures once that level was passed.

Aspartame effects on neurotransmitters levels in the brain

Aspartame affects 4 neurotransmitters levels in the brain, norepinephrine, dopamine, aspartate, serotonin and all of these can have behavioral consequences. People who are depressed have a hypersensitivity to aspartame, because it causes a disruption to the delicate balance of neurotransmitters in the brain.

One study had to be stopped because the depressed patients became more depressed while consuming the aspartame and some were becoming suicidal.

Aspartame breaks down the DNA, which will increase DNA related diseases, neurological disease and other diseases. This includes cancer and a history of having had cancer.

People who have Auto Immune disease are at higher risk especially to Lupus, which is characterized by DNA type antibodies damage.

Any of the neurogerative diseases such as Parkinson's, vascular dementia, alzheierims disease would possibly be at increased risk of worsening if they consume aspartame in high levels.

Aspartame and Multiple Sclerosis

Special concern would be anyone who has Multiple Sclerosis, or a family history of Multiple Sclerosis. MS is an inflammatory disease and it known to cause by an accumulation of excitotoxins at the site of brain damage, aspartame contains aspartic acid a known ecitotoxin.

Combining MSG and other excitotoxins greatly increase damage to the brain. It also known that the blood brain barrier is broken at the site of damage in MS Patients. And that allows anything in the blood to enter that part of the brain and worsen the damage and this is what happens when you consume aspartame.

The three components of aspartame can enter the MS legion and increase symptoms and damage. 10 % of the population has subclinical MS, they have the legion in the brain, but they don't produce outward symptoms so you don't know you have it.

A high intake of Aspartame containing foods and beverages could precipitate full blown MS cases in subclinical patients.

Aspartame can cause damage to cells and cellular structure. There is large amount of research to prove that the use of Aspartame can be very dangerous to your health.

Studies have shown the greatest risk of brain tumors are in women from aspartame breakdown formaldehyde. Recent studies have shown Aspartame to cause damage to DNA and presents harm to pregnant women and their babies. Much of the damage done to children is irreversible.

Conclusions

There are many toxins we are being intentionally exposed to. They have many far reaching physiological effects in our bodies. Many cause cancers, diabetes, obesity, brain tumors, triggers epilepsy, liver damage, DNA damage and death.

Do you want to be tricked into eating and drinking these known harmful ingredients? Did you know that we are ingesting these poisons in record amounts? Even vaccines have some of these toxins in them.

Our children and the elderly are most vulnerable, in schools, cafeterias, hospitals, restaurants and home. We deserve foods, water, milk, meat, and everything we come in contact with to be free of these deadly additives.

I have tried to raise your awareness to some of these poisons. We can fight back with our money, by not buying food and other products with these poisons in them. The FDA, EPA, and many other government agencies are not protecting us as they are being bought by corporations.

Why are we getting sick?

www.ingramcontent.com/pod-product-compliance
Lightning Source LLC
Chambersburg PA
CBHW060201290526
45789CB00003B/1108